KETOGENIC DIET COOKBOOK FOR WOMEN AFTER 50

The Complete Weight Loss Guide for Senior Women with Delicious and Easy-to-Prepare Recipes

ELIZABETH COOK

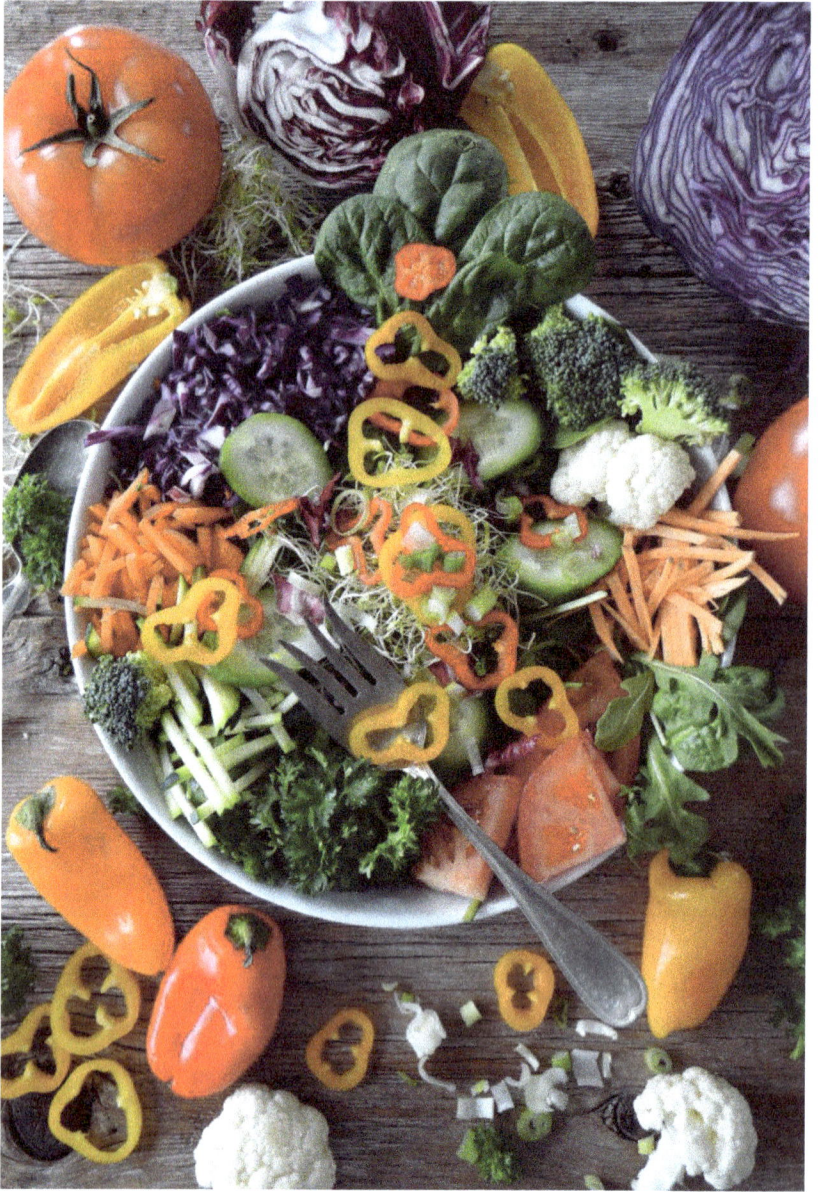

Table of Contents

Introduction

As women, when our age grows at 50, we are always looking for a quick and effective way to shed our excess weight, get our high blood sugar levels under control, reduce overall inflammation, and improve our physical and mental energy. It's frustrating to have all of these issues, especially the undeniable fats in our belly. Good thing that I found this great solution to all our worries when we reach this age level, and when our body gets weaker as time goes by. The Ketogenic diet plans.

As a woman at this age, we all know that it is much more difficult for us to lose weight than men. I have lived on a starvation level diet and exercise like a triathlete and only lose five pounds. A man will stop putting dressing on his salad and will lose twenty pounds. It just not fair. But we have the fact that we are women to blame. Women naturally have more standing between ourselves and weight loss than men do.

The mere fact that we, women, is the largest single contributor to why we find it difficult to lose weight. Since our bodies always think it needs to be prepared for a possible pregnancy, we will naturally have more body fat and less mass in our muscles than men.

Being in menopause will also cause us to add more pounds to our bodies, especially in the lower half. After menopause, our metabolism naturally slows down. Our hormones levels will decrease. These two factors alone will cause weight gain in the post-menopausal period.

There are numerous diet plan options offered to help shed weight, but the Ketogenic diet has been the most preferred lately. We've got many concerns around keto's effectiveness and exactly how to follow the diet plan in a healthy and balanced means.

The ketogenic diet for ladies at the age or over 50 is an easy and ideal way to shed extra pounds, stay energetic, and enjoy a healthy life. It does not only balances hormones but also improves our body capabilities without causing any harm to our overall wellness. Thus, if you are fighting with post-menopausal symptoms and other health issues, you should do a Keto diet right away!

A Keto diet is a lifestyle, not a diet so, treat it like the same. The best way to approach keto to gain maximum benefits, especially for women over 50s, is to treat it as a lifestyle. You can't restrict your meal intake through obstructive and strict diets forever, right? It's the fundamental reason fad diets fail — we limit ourselves from too much to get rapid results, then we're are right back again at the weight where we started, or God forbid worse.

Keto is not a kind of diet that can be followed strictly forever — unless you need it as a therapeutic diet (i.e., epilepsy), a very narrow category. In keto diet, we slowly transit into a curative state that we can withstand forever in a healthier way.

So, for me, being on a keto diet does not mean that I will be in ketosis forever. Instead, it means letting myself love consideration, such as a few desserts while vacationing or partying. It does not set me back to enjoy these desserts and let me consider it as the end of the diet. I can wake up the following morning and go back to the keto lifestyle, most suitable for me and my body consistently.

It allows my body to boost its fat loss drastically in many cases, which helps in decreasing pockets of undesirable fat.

With Keto Diet, it's not only giving weight loss assistance to reduce my weight, yet it can likewise ward off yearnings for unhealthy foods and protect me against calories collisions throughout the day. That is why I want it to share with you how promising this Keto diet. As our age grow older, we must not let our body do the same. Focus your mindset on this fantastic diet, read, apply, and enjoy its best benefits.

© Copyright 2020 by Elizabeth Cook - All rights reserved.

The following Book is reproduced below with the goal of providing information that is as accurate and reliable as possible. Regardless, purchasing this Book can be seen as consent to the fact that both the publisher and the author of this book are in no way experts on the topics discussed within and that any recommendations or suggestions that are made herein are for entertainment purposes only. Professionals should be consulted as needed prior to undertaking any of the action endorsed herein.

This declaration is deemed fair and valid by both the American Bar Association and the Committee of Publishers Association and is legally binding throughout the United States.

Furthermore, the transmission, duplication, or reproduction of any of the following work including specific information will be considered an illegal act irrespective of if it is done electronically or in print. This extends to creating a secondary or tertiary copy of the work or a recorded copy and is only allowed with the express written consent from the Publisher. All additional right reserved.

The information in the following pages is broadly considered a truthful and accurate account of facts and as such, any inattention, use, or misuse of the information in question by the reader will render any resulting actions solely under their purview. There are no scenarios in which the publisher or the original author of this work can be in any fashion deemed liable for any hardship or damages that may befall them after undertaking information described herein.

Additionally, the information in the following pages is intended only for informational purposes and should thus be thought of as universal. As befitting its nature, it is presented without assurance regarding its prolonged validity or interim quality. Trademarks that are mentioned are done without written consent and can in no way be considered an endorsement from the trademark holder.

Breakfast Recipes

1.   Southwest Scrambled Egg Bites

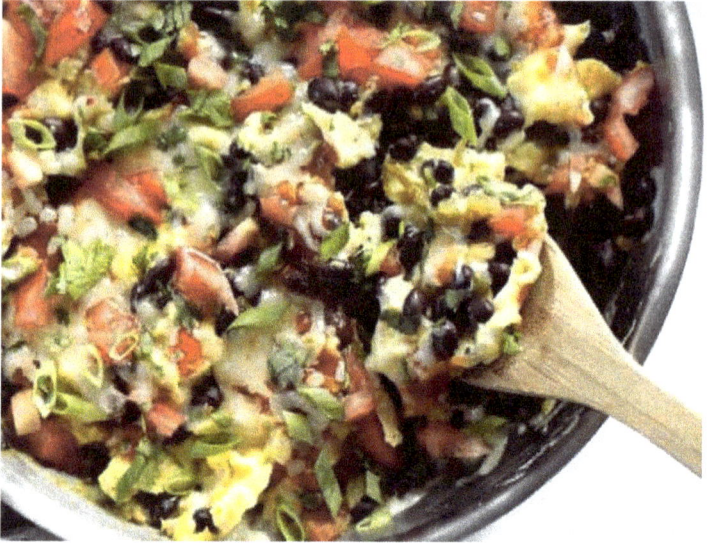

Preparation time: 10 minutes

Cooking time: 23 minutes

Servings: 4

Ingredients:

- 5 eggs

- 1/2 teaspoon hot pepper sauce

- 1/3 cup tomatoes

- 3 tablespoons green chilies

- 1 teaspoon black pepper

- 1/2 teaspoon salt

- 2 tablespoons nondairy milk

Directions:

1. Mix both the eggs and milk in a large cup. Add the hot sauce, pepper, and salt. Put a small diced chilies and diced tomatoes in silicone cups.

2. Fill each with 3/4 full with the egg mixture.

3. Put the trivet in the pot and pour 1 cup water. Put the mold on the trivet. Set to high for 8 minutes. Cool down before serving.

Nutrition:

Calories: 106

Carbs: 2g

Protein: 7.5g

Fats: 7.4g

2.   Omelet Bites

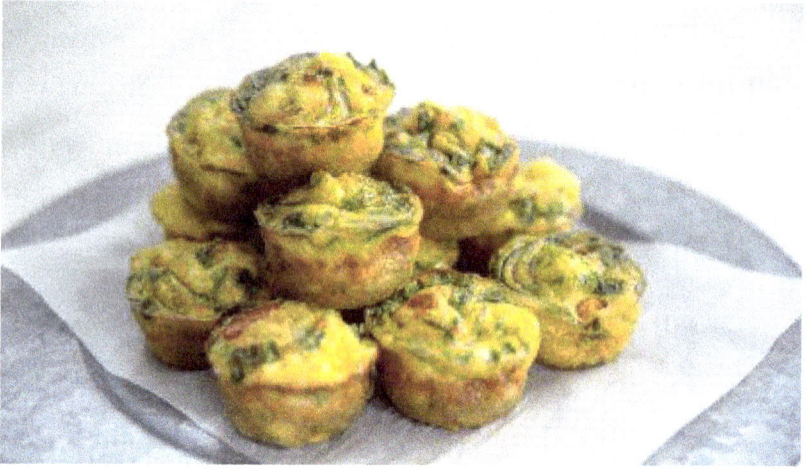

Preparation time: 5 minutes

Cooking time: 8 minutes

Servings: 3

Ingredients:

- 1 handful mushrooms
- green onion
- green peppers
- 1/8 teaspoon hot sauce
- Pepper, salt, mustard, garlic powder
- 1/2 cup cheese cheddar
- 1/2 cup cheese cottage
- 2 deli ham slices
- 4 eggs

Directions:

1. Whisk eggs, then the cheddar and cottage. Put the ham, veggies, and seasonings; mix. Pour the mixture into greased silicone molds.

2. Put the trivet with the molds in the pot then fill with 2 cups water. Steam for about 8 minutes.

Nutrition:

Calories: 260

Carbs: 6g

Protein: 22g

Fats: 16g

3.   Avocado Pico Egg Bites

Preparation time: 15 minutes

Cooking time: 10 minutes

Servings: 7

Ingredients:

- Egg bites:
- 1/ cup cheese cottage
- 1/2 cup cheese Mexican blend
- 1/4 cup cream heavy cream
- 1/4 teaspoon chili powder
- 1/4 teaspoon cumin
- 1/4 teaspoon garlic powder
- 4 eggs
- Pepper
- salt
- Pico de Gallo:
- 1 avocado
- 1 jalapeno
- 1/2 teaspoon salt
- 1/4 onion
- 2 tablespoons cilantro

- 2 teaspoons lime juice

- 4 Roma tomatoes

Directions:

1. Mix all of the Pico de Gallo fixing except for the avocado. Gently fold in the avocado.

2. Blend all the egg bites ingredients in a blender. Spoon 1 tablespoon of Pico de Gallo into each egg bite silicone mold.

3. Place the trivet in the pot then fill with 1 cup water. Put the molds in the trivet. Set to high within 10 minutes. Remove. Serve topped with cheese and Pico de Gallo.

Nutrition:

Calories: 118

Carbs: 1g

Protein: 7g

Fats: 9g

4. Salmon Scramble

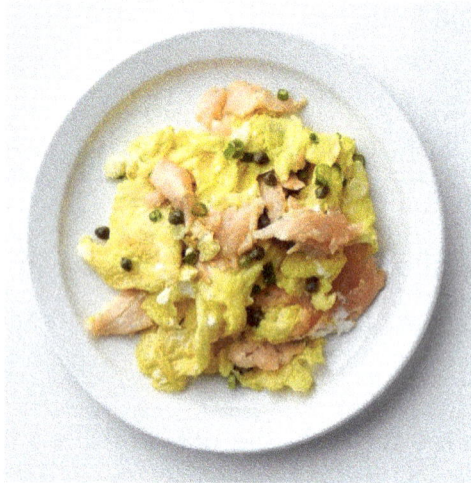

Preparation time: 10 minutes

Cooking time: 5 minutes

Servings: 1

Ingredients:

- 2 smoked salmon pieces
- 1 organic egg yolk
- 1/8 teaspoon. red pepper flakes
- Black pepper
- 2 organic eggs
- 1 tablespoon. dill
- 1/8 teaspoon. garlic powder
- 1 tablespoon. olive oil

Directions:

1. Beat all items except salmon and oil. Stir in chopped salmon. Warm-up oil over medium-low heat in a frying pan. Add the egg mixture and cook within 3-5 minutes. Serve.

Nutrition:

Calories: 376

Carbs: 3.4g

Protein: 24g

Fats: 24.8g

5. Cheddar & Bacon Egg Bites

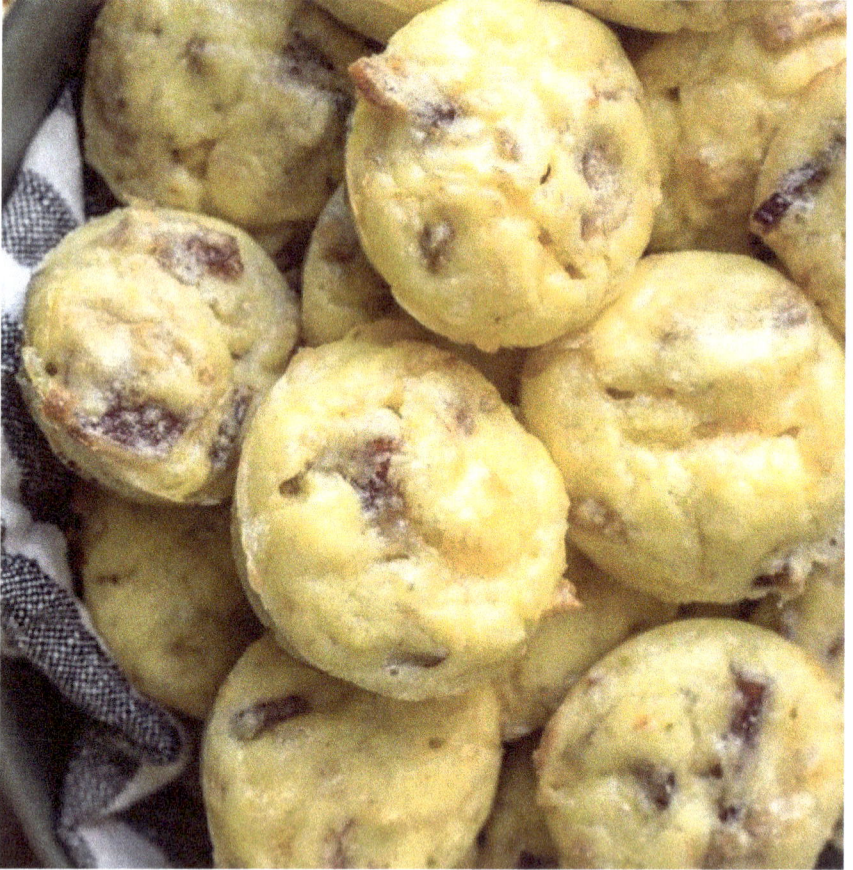

Preparation time: 10 minutes

Cooking time: 8 minutes

Servings: 7

Ingredients:

- 1 cup sharp cheddar cheese

- 1 tablespoon parsley flakes

- 4 eggs

- 4 tablespoons cream

- Hot sauce

- 1 cup of water

- 1/2 cup cheese

- 4 slices bacon

Directions:

1. Blend the cream, cheddar, cottage, and egg in the blender; 30 seconds. Stir in the parsley. Grease silicone egg bite molds.

2. Divide the crumbled bacon between them. Put the egg batter into each cup. With a piece of foil, cover each mold.

3. Place the trivet with the molds in the pot then fill with 1 cup water. Steam for 8 minutes. Remove, let rest for 5 minutes.

4. Serve, sprinkled with black pepper and optional hot sauce.

Nutrition:

Calories: 167

Carbs: 1.5g

Protein: 13.5g

Fats: 11.7g

6.   Mexican Scrambled Eggs

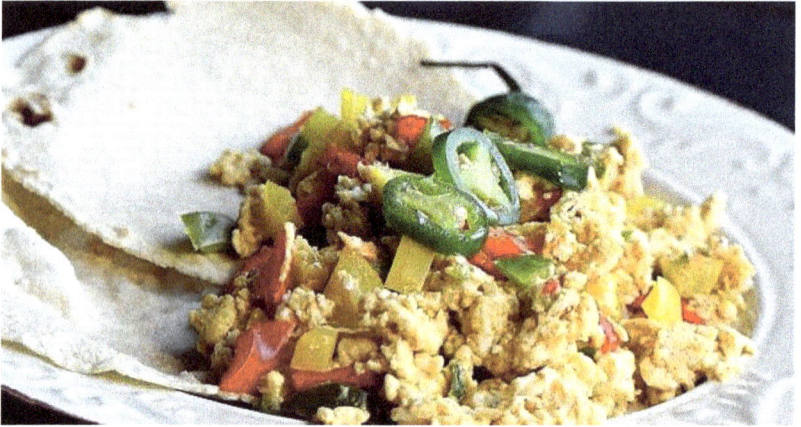

Preparation time: 5 minutes

Cooking time: 10 minutes

Servings: 6

Ingredients:

- 6 Eggs

- 2 Jalapeños

- 1 Tomato

- 3 oz. Cheese

- 2 tablespoon. Butter

Directions:

1. Warm-up butter over medium heat in a large pan. Add tomatoes, jalapeños, and green onions then cook within 3 minutes.

2. Add eggs, and continue within 2 minutes. Add cheese and season to taste. Serve.

Nutrition:

Calories: 239

Carbs: 2.38g

Protein: 13.92g

Fats: 19.32g

7. Bacon Egg Bites

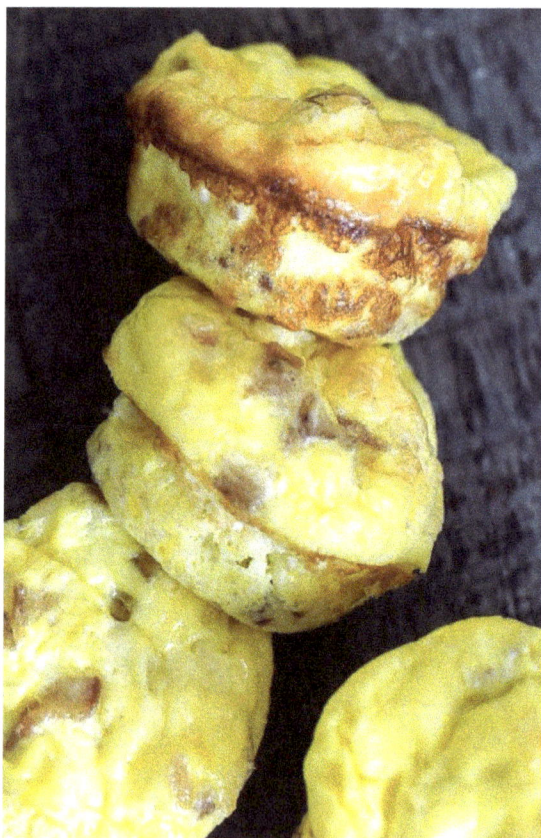

Preparation time: 10 minutes

Cooking time: 22 minutes

Servings: 9

Ingredients:

- 1 cup cheese

- 1/2 green pepper

- 1/2 cup cottage cheese

- 4 slices bacon

- Pepper

- salt

- 1 cup red onion

- 1 cup of water

- 1/4 cup whip cream

- 1/4 cup egg whites

- 4 eggs

Directions:

1. Blend egg whites, eggs, cream, cheese (cottage), shredded cheese, pepper, and salt within 30 to 45 seconds in a blender. Put the egg mixture into mini muffin cups.

2. Top each with bacon, peppers, and onion. Cover the muffin cups tightly with foil. Place the trivet in the pot and pour 1 cup water.

3. Put the cups on the trivet. Set to steam for 12 minutes.

Nutrition:

Calories: 124

Carbs: 3g

Protein: 9g

Fats: 8

8.   Caprese Omelet

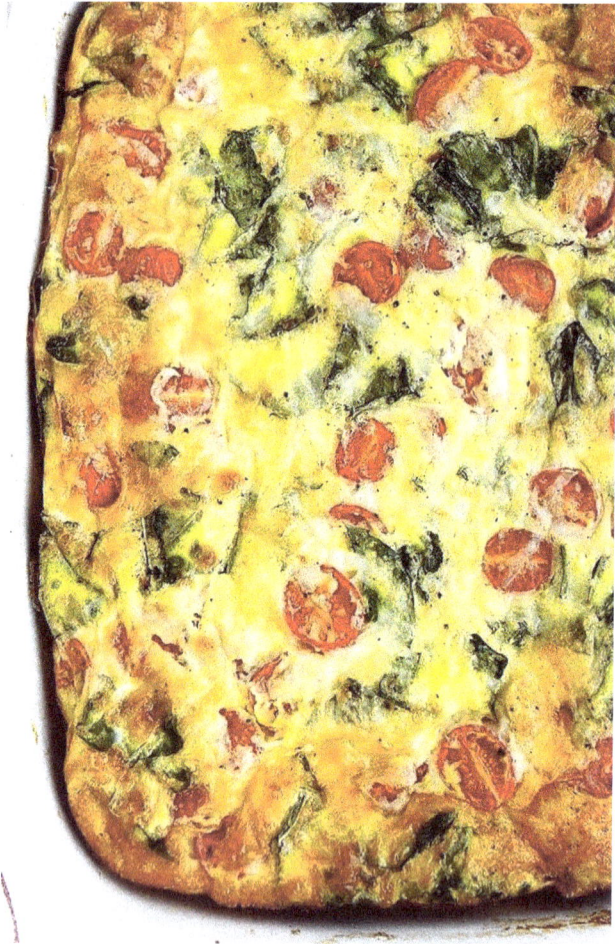

Preparation time: 10 minutes

Cooking time: 10 minutes

Servings: 2

Ingredients:

- 6 eggs

- Olive oil 2 tablespoon.

- Halved cherry tomatoes 3½ oz.

- Dried basil 1 tablespoon.

- Mozzarella cheese 5 1/3 oz.

Directions:

1. Mix the basil, eggs, salt and black pepper in a bowl. Place a large skillet with oil over medium heat. Once hot, add tomatoes and cook.

2. Top with egg and cook. Add cheese, adjust heat to low, and allow to set before serving fully.

Nutrition:

Calories: 423

Carbs: 6.81g

Protein: 43.08g

Fats: 60.44g

9.   Sausage Omelet

Preparation time: 10 minutes

Cooking time: 15 minutes

Servings: 2

Ingredients:

- ½ pound gluten-free sausage links
- ½ cup heavy whipping cream
- Salt
- black pepper
- 8 large organic eggs
- 1 cup cheddar cheese
- ¼ teaspoon. red pepper flakes

Directions:

1. Warm-up oven to 350°F. Grease a baking dish. Cook the sausage within 8–10 minutes.

2. Put the rest of the fixing in a bowl and beat. Remove sausage from the heat.

3. Place cooked sausage in the baking dish then top with the egg mixture. Bake within 30 minutes. Slice and serve.

Nutrition:

Calories: 334

Carbs: 1.1g

Protein: 20.6g

Fats: 27.3g

10. Brown Hash with Zucchini

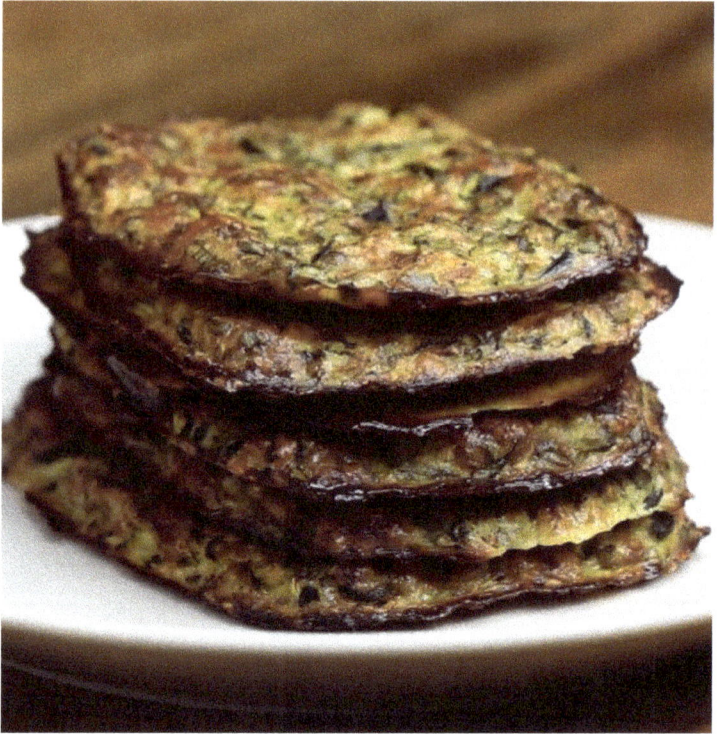

Preparation time: 10 minutes

Cooking time: 20 minutes

Servings: 2

Ingredients:

- 1 small onion

- 6 to 8 mushrooms

- 2 Cups grass-fed ground beef

- 1 Pinch salt

- 1 Pinch ground black pepper

- ½ teaspoon smoked paprika

- 2 eggs

- 1 avocado

- 10 black olives

Directions:

1. Warm-up air fryer for 350° F. Grease a pan with coconut oil. Add the onions, the mushrooms, the salt plus pepper to the pan.

2. Add the ground beef and the smoked paprika and eggs. Mix, then place the pan in Air Fryer. Set to cook within 18 to 20 minutes with a temperature, 375° F.

3. Serve with chopped parsley and diced avocado!

Nutrition:

Calories: 290

Carbs: 15g

Protein: 20g

Fats: 23g

Lunch Recipes

11.   Keto Chicken Club Lettuce Wrap

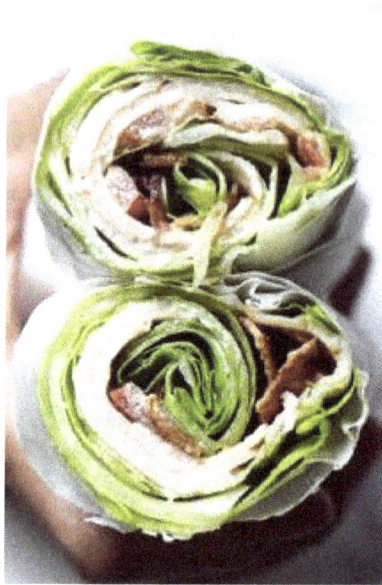

Preparation Time: 15 minutes

Cooking Time: 15 minutes

Servings: 1

Ingredients:

- 1 head iceberg lettuce
- 1 tablespoon. mayonnaise
- 6 slices of organic chicken
- Bacon
- Tomato

Directions:

1. Layer 6-8 large leaves of lettuce in the center of the parchment paper, around 9-10 inches.

2. Spread the mayo in the center and lay with chicken, bacon, and tomato.

3. Roll the wrap halfway through, then roll tuck in the ends of the wrap.

4. Cut it in half. Serve.

Nutrition:

Net carbs: 4g

Fiber: 2g

Fat: 78g

Protein: 28g

Calories: 837

12. Keto Broccoli Salad

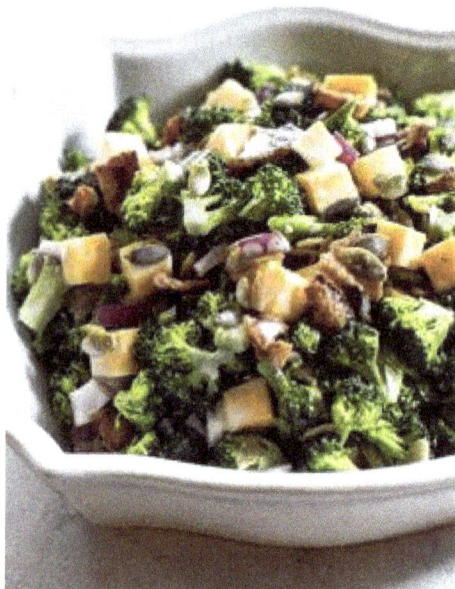

Preparation Time: 10 minutes

Cooking Time: 0 minutes

Servings: 4-6

Ingredients:

For salad

- 2 Broccoli

- 2 Red Cabbage

- .5 c Sliced Almonds

- 1 Green Onions

- .5 c Raisins

For the orange almond dressing

- .33 c Orange Juice

- .25 c Almond Butter

- 2 tablespoon Coconut Aminos

- 1 Shallot

- Salt

Directions:

1. Pulse the salt, shallot, amino, nut butter, and orange juice using a blender.

2. Combine other fixing in a bowl. Toss it with dressing and serve.

Nutrition:

Net carbs: 13g

Fiber: 0g

Fat: 94g

Protein: 22g

Calories: 1022

13.   Keto Sheet Pan Chicken and Rainbow Veggies

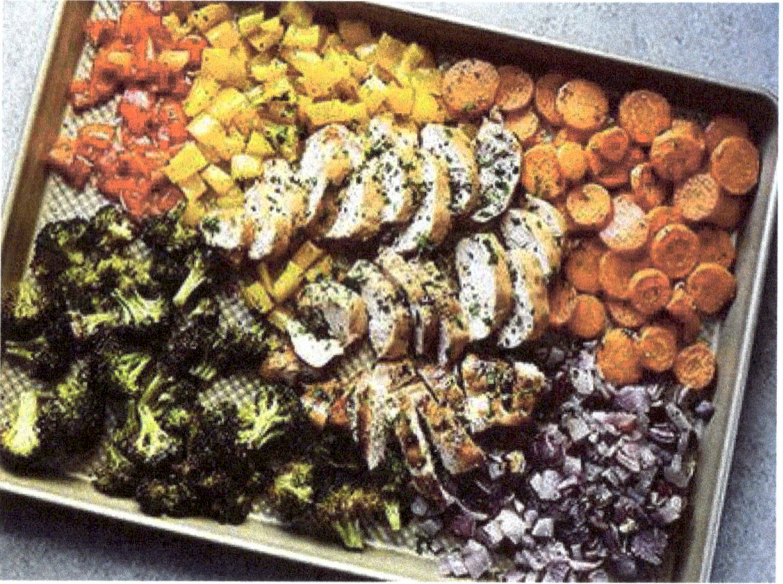

Preparation Time: 15 minutes

Cooking Time: 25 minutes

Servings: 4

Ingredients:

- Nonstick spray

- 1-pound Chicken Breasts

- 1 tablespoon Sesame Oil

- 2 tablespoon Soy Sauce

- 2 tablespoon Honey

- 2 Red Pepper

- 2 Yellow Pepper

- 3 Carrots

- ½ Broccoli

- 2 Red Onions

- 2 tablespoon EVOO

- Pepper & salt

- .25 c Parsley

Directions:

1. Grease the baking sheet, warm-up the oven to a temperature of 400-degrees.

2. Put the chicken in the middle of the sheet. Separately, combine the oil and the soy sauce. Brush over the chicken.

3. Separate veggies across the plate. Sprinkle with oil and then toss. Put pepper & salt.

4. Set tray into the oven and cook within 25 minutes. Garnish using parsley. Serve.

Nutrition:

Net carbs: 9g

Fiber: 0g

Fat: 30g

Protein: 30g

Calories: 437kcal

14. Cole Slaw Keto Wrap

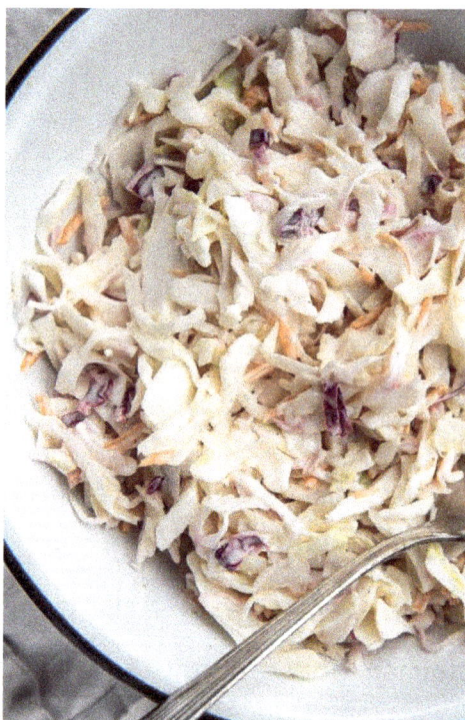

Preparation Time: 15 minutes

Cooking Time: 0 minutes

Servings: 2

Ingredients:

- 3 c Red Cabbage

- .5 c Green Onions

- .75 c Mayo

- 2 teaspoon Apple Cider Vinegar

- .25 teaspoon Salt

- 16 pcs Collard Green

- 1-pound Ground Meat, cooked

- .33 c Alfalfa Sprouts

-         Toothpicks

Directions:

1. Mix slaw items with a spoon in a large-sized bowl.

2. Place a collard green on a plate and scoop a tablespoon of coleslaw on the edge of the leaf. Top it with a scoop of meat and sprouts. Roll and tuck the sides.

3. Insert the toothpicks. Serve.

Nutrition:

Calories: 409

Net carbs: 4g

Fiber: 2g

Fat: 42g

Protein: 2g

15.   Keto Caesar Salad

Preparation Time: 15 minutes

Cooking Time: 0 minutes

Servings: 4

Ingredients:

- Cups Mayonnaise
- 3 tablespoons Apple Cider Vinegar
- 1 teaspoon Dijon Mustard
- 4 Anchovy Fillets
- 24 Romaine Heart Leaves
- 4 oz Pork Rinds
- Parmesan

Directions:

1. Process the mayo with ACV, mustard, and anchovies into a blender. Prepare romaine leaves and pour the dressing. Top with pork rinds and serve.

Nutrition:

Net carbs: 4g

Fiber: 3g

Fat: 86g

Protein: 47g

Calories: 993kcal

16.   Skinny Bang-Bang Zucchini Noodles

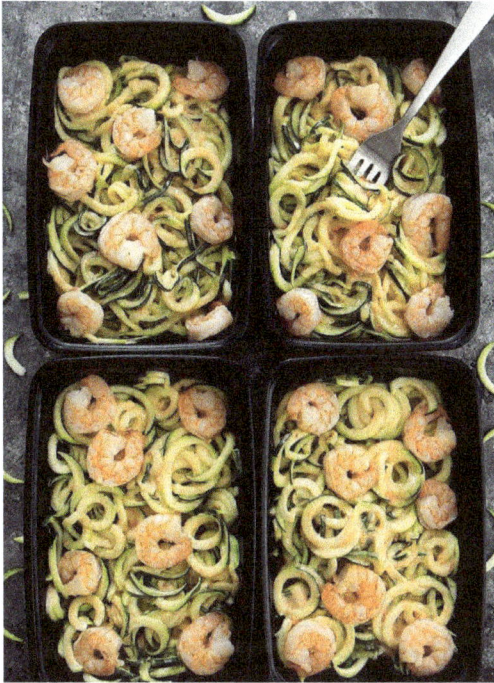

Preparation Time: 15 minutes

Cooking Time: 15 minutes

Servings: 4

Ingredients:

For the noodles

- 4 medium zucchinis spiraled

- 1 tablespoon. olive oil

For the sauce

- 0.25 cup + 2 tablespoons Plain Greek Yogurt

- 0.25 cup + 2 tablespoons Mayo

- 0.25 cup + 2 tablespoons Thai Sweet Chili Sauce

- Teaspoons Honey

- Teaspoons Sriracha

- 2 teaspoons Lime Juice

Directions:

1. Pour the oil into a large skillet at medium temperature. Stir in the spiraled zucchini noodles. Cook.

2. Remove then drain, and let it rest 10 minutes. Combine sauce items into a bowl.

3. Mix in the noodles to the sauce. Serve.

Nutrition:

Net carbs: 18g

Fiber: 0g

Fat: 1g

Protein: 9g

Calories: 161g

17.   Keto Bacon Sushi

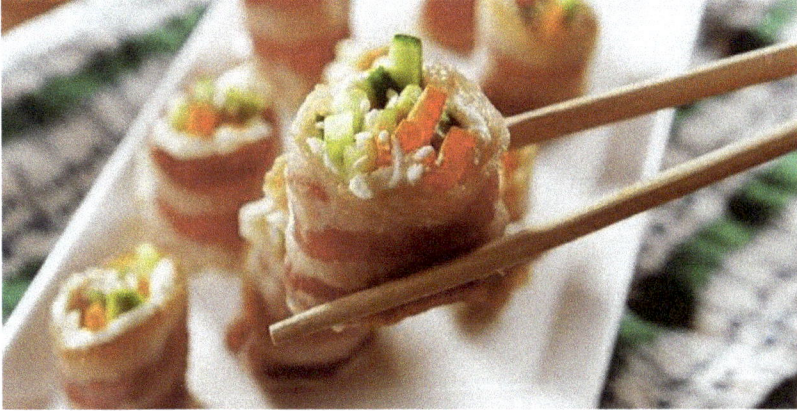

Preparation time: 15 minutes

Cooking time: 13 minutes

Servings: 4

Ingredients:

- Six slices bacon

- One avocado

- Two Persian cucumbers

- Two medium carrots

- Four oz. cream cheese

Directions:

1. Warm-up oven to 400F. Line a baking sheet. Place bacon halves in an even layer and bake, 11 to 13 minutes.

2. Meanwhile, slice cucumbers, avocado, and carrots into parts roughly the width of the bacon.

3. Spread an even layer of cream cheese in the cooled down bacon. Divide vegetables evenly and place it on one end. Roll up vegetables tightly. Garnish and serve.

Nutrition:

11 g carbohydrates

28g protein

30g fat

18.   Chicken Wings and Blue Cheese Dressing

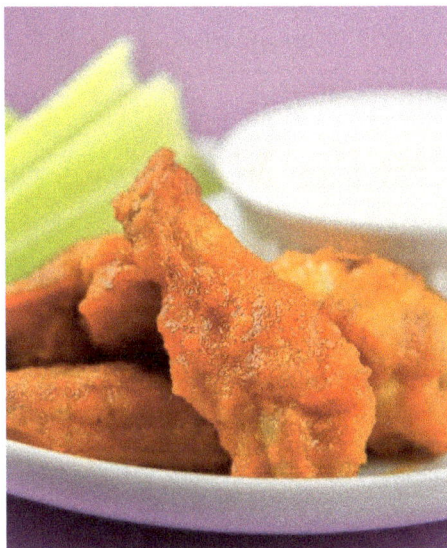

Preparation Time: 70 minutes

Cooking Time: 25 minutes

Servings: 4

Ingredients:

- One-third cup mayonnaise
- One-fourth cup sour cream
- Three teaspoon. lemon juice
- One-fourth teaspoon. of each:
- Salt
- Garlic powder
- Half cup whipping cream

- Three ounces blue cheese

For the chicken wings:

- Two pounds chicken wings
- Two tablespoons. olive oil
- One-fourth teaspoon. garlic powder
- One clove garlic
- One-third teaspoon. black pepper
- One teaspoon. salt
- Two ounces parmesan cheese

Directions:

1. Mix all the blue cheese dressing items in a bowl. Chill within forty minutes.
2. Combine the chicken with olive oil and spices. Marinate for thirty minutes.
3. Bake in the oven for twenty-five minutes. Toss the chicken wings with parmesan cheese in a bowl.
4. Serve with blue cheese dressing by the side.

Nutrition:

Calories: 839.3

Protein: 51.2g

Carbs: 2.9g

Fat: 67.8g - Fiber: 0.2g

19. Salmon Burgers with Lemon Butter and Mash

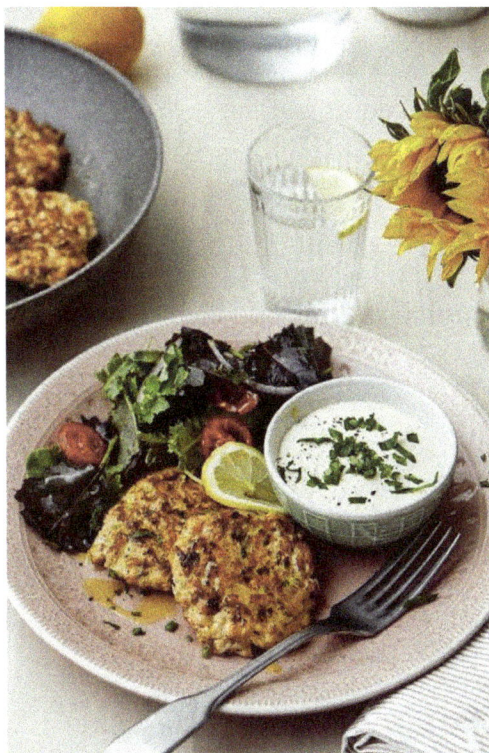

Preparation Time: 70 minutes

Cooking Time: 15 minutes

Servings: 4

Ingredients:

For the salmon burgers:

- Two pounds salmon
- One egg
- Half yellow onion

- One teaspoon. salt
- Half teaspoon. black pepper
- Two ounces butter
- For the green mash:
- One-pound broccoli
- Five ounces of butter
- Two ounces parmesan cheese
- Pepper
- salt

For the lemon butter:

- Four ounces butter
- Two tablespoons. lemon juice
- Pepper
- salt

Directions:

1. Warm-up your oven at 100 degrees.
2. Cut the salmon into small pieces. Combine all the burger items with the fish in a blender. Pulse for thirty seconds. Make eight patties.
3. Warm-up butter in an iron skillet. Fry the burgers for five minutes.

4. Boil water, along with some salt in a pot, put the broccoli florets. Cook for three to four minutes. Drain. Add parmesan cheese and butter. Blend the ingredients using an immersion blender. Add pepper and salt.

5. Combine lemon juice with butter, pepper, and salt. Beat using an electric beater.

6. Put a dollop of lemon butter on the top and green mash by the side. Serve.

Nutrition:

Calories: 1025.3

Protein: 44.5g

Carbs: 6.8g

Fat: 90.1g

Fiber: 3.1g

20. Egg Salad Recipe

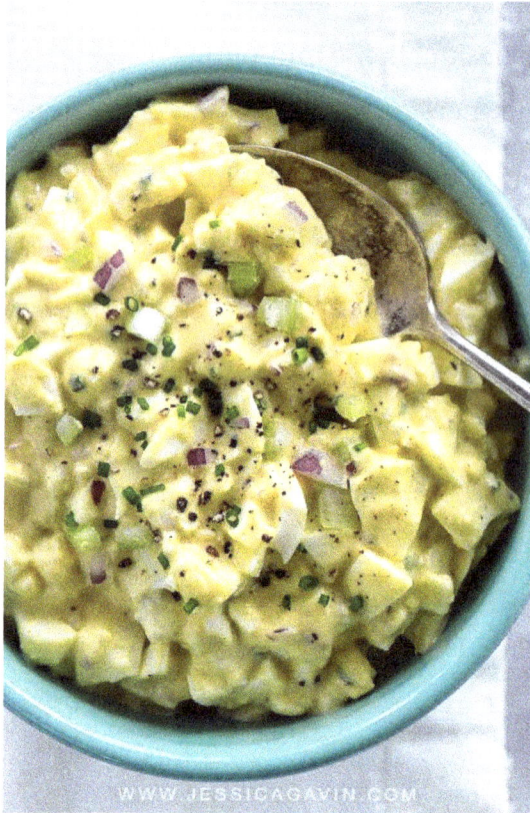

Preparation Time: 15 minutes

Cooking Time: 20 minutes

Servings: 6

Ingredients:

- 3 tablespoon. mayonnaise

- 3 tablespoon. Greek yogurt

- 2 tablespoon. red wine vinegar

- Kosher salt

- ground black pepper

- Eight hard-boiled eggs

- Eight strips bacon

- One avocado

- 1/2 c. crumbled blue cheese

- 1/2 c. cherry tomatoes

- 2 tablespoon. chives

Directions:

1. Stir mayonnaise, cream, and the red wine vinegar in a small bowl put pepper and salt.

2. Mix the eggs, bacon, avocado, blue cheese, and cherry tomatoes in a large bowl. Fold in the mayonnaise dressing put salt and pepper. Garnish with the chives and serve.

Nutrition:

Calories: 200

Carbs: 3g

Fat: 18g

Protein: 10g

SNACKS AND CAKES

21. Spicy Crab Dip

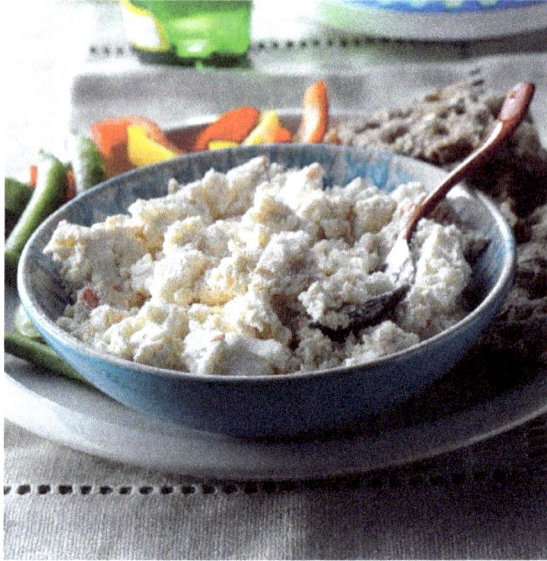

Preparation Time: 15 minutes

Cooking Time: 20 minutes

Servings: 3

Ingredients:

- 8 oz cream cheese

- 1 tablespoon. onions

- 1 tablespoon. lemon juice

- 2 tablespoon. Worcestershire sauce

- 1/8 teaspoon. t. black

- Cayenne pepper

- 2 tablespoon. milk

- 6 oz crabmeat

Directions:

1. Warm-up oven to 375 ° F.

2. Pour the cream cheese into a bowl. Add the onions, lemon juice, Worcestershire sauce, black pepper, and cayenne pepper. Mix. Stir in the milk and crab meat.

3. Cook uncovered within 15 minutes. Serve.

Nutrition:

Calories: 134 Carbs: 4g

Fat: 12g Protein: 4g

22.   Potatoes" of Parmesan cheese

Preparation Time: 15 minutes

Cooking Time: 10 minutes

Servings: 3

Ingredients:

- 75 g Parmesan cheese
- 1 tablespoon Chia seeds
- 2 tablespoon whole flaxseeds
- 2½ tablespoon pumpkin seeds

Directions:

1. Warm-up oven to 180 ° C.
2. Combine both the cheese and seeds in a bowl.
3. Put small piles of the mixture on the baking paper, bake within 8 to 10 minutes
4. Remove and serve.

Nutrition:

Calories: 165

Carbs: 18g

Fat: 9g

Protein: 3g

23. Chili Cheese Chicken with Crispy and Delicious Cabbage Salad

Preparation Time: 15 minutes

Cooking Time: 70 minutes

Servings: 5

Ingredients:

- Chili Cheese Chicken
- 400 grams of chicken
- 200 grams tomatoes
- 100 grams of cream cheese
- 125 grams cheddar
- 40 grams jalapenos
- 60 grams of bacon
- Crispy Cabbage Salad
- 0.5 pcs casserole
- 200 grams Brussels sprouts
- 2 grams of almonds
- 3 paragraph mandarins
- 1 tablespoon olive oil
- 1 teaspoon apple cider vinegar
- 0.5 teaspoon salt

- 0.25 teaspoon pepper

- 1 tablespoon lemon

Directions:

1. Warm-up oven at 200 °. Put tomatoes half in the bottom of a baking dish. Put chicken fillets, half cream cheese on each chicken fillet, and sprinkle with cheddar.

2. Spread jalapenos and bake within 25 minutes. Place bacon on a baking sheet with baking paper, and bake within 10 minutes.

3. For cabbage salad:

4. Blend the Brussels sprouts and cumin in a food processor.

5. Make the dressing of juice from one mandarin, olive oil, apple cider vinegar, salt, pepper, and lemon juice.

6. Put the cabbage in a dish and spread the dressing over. Chop almonds, cut the tangerine into slices and place it on the salad. Sprinkle the bacon over the chicken dish. Serve.

Nutrition:

Calories: 515

Carbs: 35g

Fat: 23g

Protein: 42g

24.   Keto Pumpkin Pie Sweet and Spicy

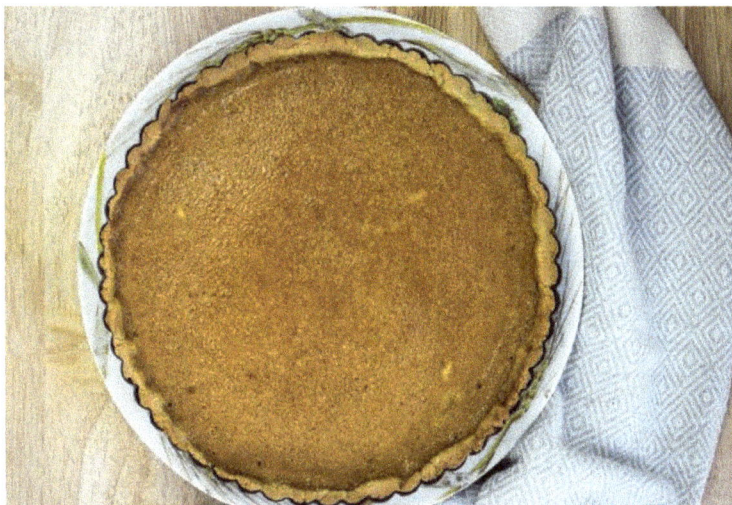

Preparation Time: 15 minutes

Cooking Time: 60 minutes

Servings: 5

Ingredients:

Pie Bottom

- 110 grams of almond flour
- 50 grams serine
- 0.5 teaspoon salt
- 1 scoop protein powder
- 1 paragraph eggs
- 80 grams of butter
- 15 grams of fiber

The Filling

- 1 pcs Hokkaido
- 3 paragraph egg yolks
- 60 ml of coconut fat
- 1 teaspoon vanilla powder
- 15 grams of protein powder
- 1 teaspoon cinnamon
- 2 grams sucrine
- 0.5 teaspoon cardamom Bla
- 0.5 teaspoon cloves

Directions:

1. Warm-up oven to 175 °.
2. Combine all the dry fixing and add the wet ones. Mix and shape it into a dough lump. Put in a baking paper, then flatten the dough. Prick holes then bake within 8-10 minutes.
3. For filling:
4. Cut the meat of Hokkaido and cook within 15-20 minutes. Process it with the other fixing. Pour the stuffing into the baked pie and bake again within 25-30 minutes. Cool and serve.

Nutrition:

Calories: 229

Carbs: 4g

Fat: 22g

Protein: 8g

25. Blackened Tilapia with Zucchini Noodles

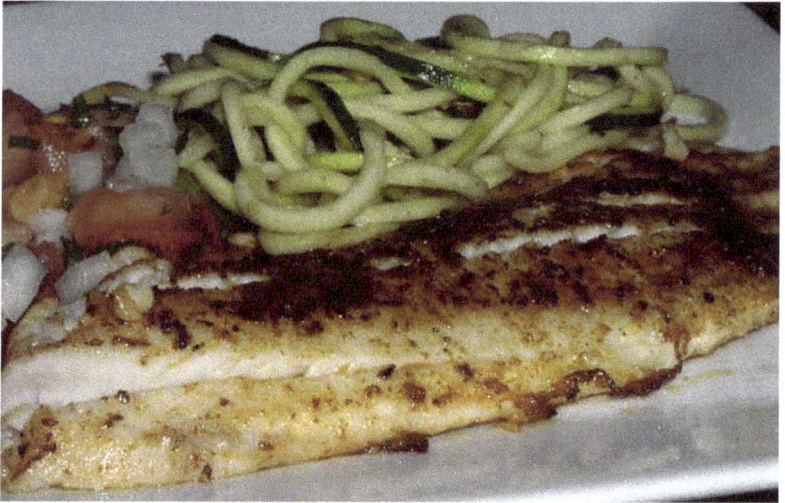

Preparation Time: 15 minutes

Cooking Time: 10 minutes

Servings: 5

Ingredients:

2 zucchinis

¾ teaspoon salt

2 garlic cloves

1 cup Pico de Gallo

1 ½ pounds fish

2 teaspoons olive oil

½ teaspoon cumin

¼ teaspoon garlic powder

½ paprika

½ teaspoon pepper

Directions:

Mix half salt, pepper, cumin, paprika, and garlic powder, rub to the fish thoroughly. Cook within 3 minutes each side and remove it. Cook zucchini and garlic, remaining salt within 2 minutes. Serve.

Nutrition:

Calories: 220

Carbs: 27g

Fat: 2g

Protein: 24g

26. Bell Pepper Nachos

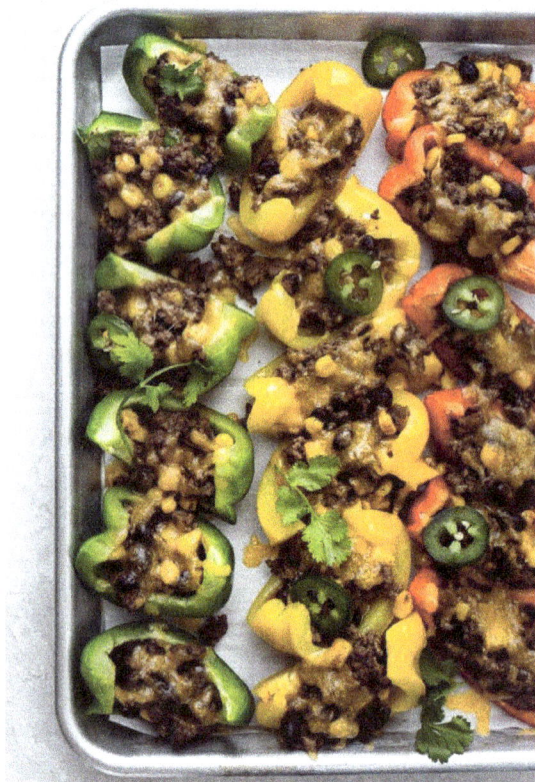

Preparation Time: 15 minutes

Cooking Time: 10 minutes

Servings: 2

Ingredients:

- 2 bell peppers
- 4 ounces beef ground
- ¼ teaspoon cumin
- ¼ cup guacamole

- salt

- 1 cup cheese

- ¼ teaspoon chili powder

- 1 tablespoon vegetable oil

- 2 tablespoons sour cream

- ¼ cup Pico de Gallo

Directions:

1. Put the bell peppers in a microwave dish, sprinkle salt and splash water on it and microwave within 4 minutes and cut it in 4 pieces.

2. Toast the chili powder and cumin in the pan for 30 seconds. Put the salted beef, stir and cook within 4 minutes.

3. Put on all the pieces of pepper. Add cheese and cook within 1 minute. Serve with Pico de Gallo, guacamole, and cream.

Nutrition:

Calories: 475

Carbs: 19g

Fat: 24g

Protein: 50g

27. Radish, Carrot & Cilantro Salad

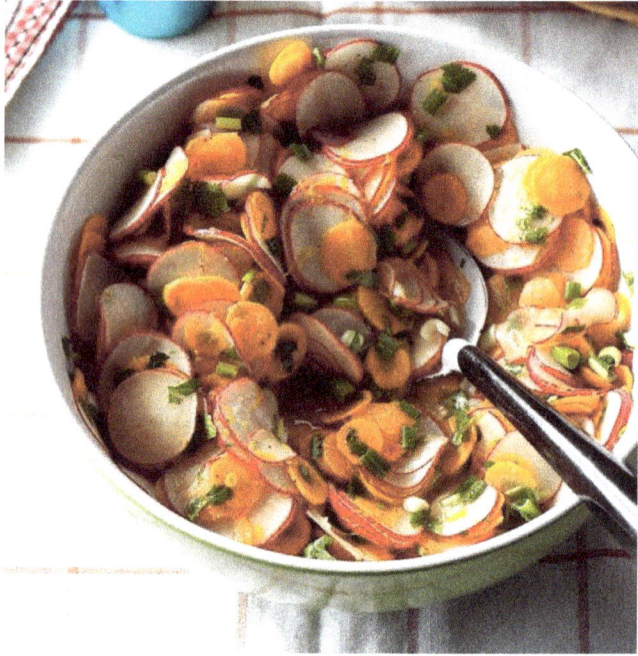

Preparation Time: 15 minutes

Cooking Time: 0 minutes

Servings: 2

Ingredients:

- 1 ½ pounds carrots

- ¼ cup cilantro

- 1 ½ pound radish

- ½ teaspoon salt

- 6 onions

- ¼ teaspoon black pepper

- 3 tablespoons lemon juice

- 3 tablespoons orange juice

- 2 tablespoons olive oil

Directions:

1. Mix all the items until they merged adequately. Chill and serve.

Nutrition:

Calories: 33 Carbs: 7g

Fat: 0g Protein: 0g

28. Asparagus-Mushroom Frittata

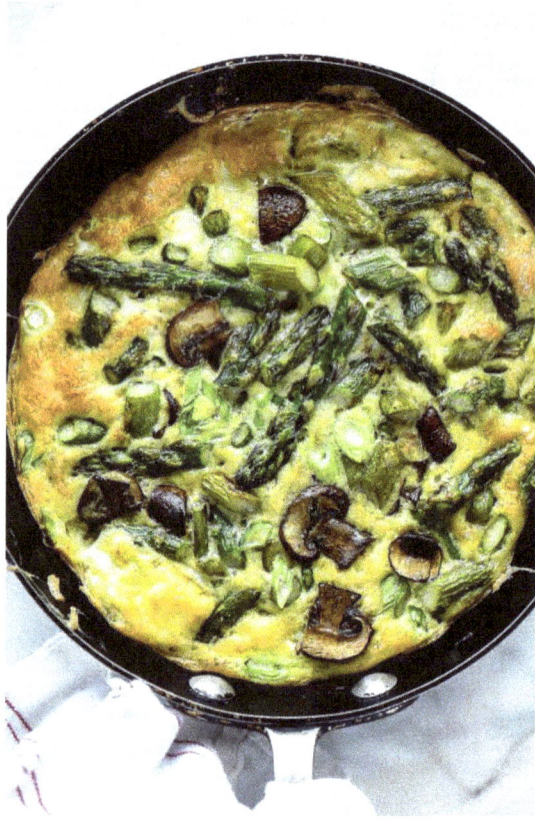

Preparation Time: 15 minutes

Cooking Time: 25 minutes

Servings: 2

Ingredients:

- 1 tablespoon olive oil
- 1garlic clove
- ¼ cup onion
- 2 cups button mushrooms

- 1 asparagus

- 1 tablespoon thyme

- 6 eggs

- ½ cup feta cheese

- salt

- black pepper

Directions:

1. Cook onions within 5 minutes. Put mushroom plus garlic then cook within 5 minutes. Mix thyme, salt, pepper, and asparagus and cook within 3 minutes.

2. Beat eggs and cheese in a bowl and pour it in the pan and cook for 2 to 3 minutes. Bake within 10 minutes.

Nutrition:

Calories: 129

Carbs: 2g

Fat: 7g

Protein: 9g

29. Shrimp Avocado Salad

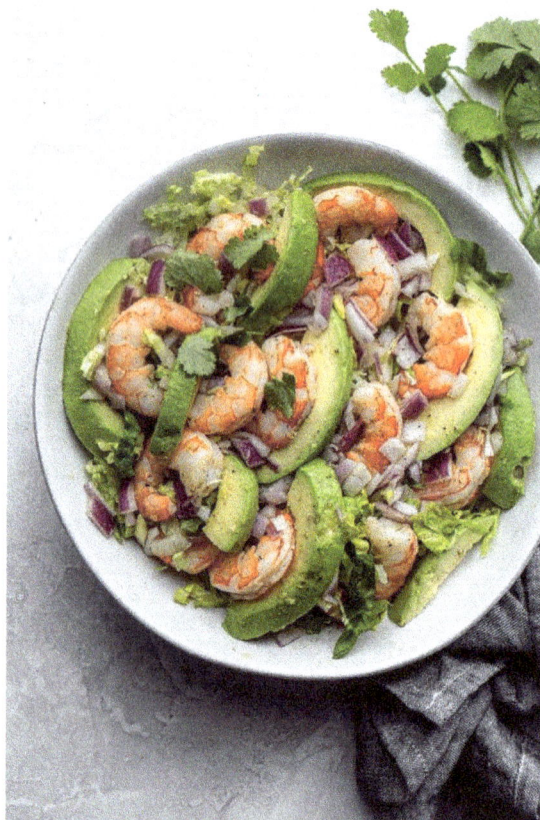

Preparation Time: 15 minutes

Cooking Time: 0 minutes

Servings: 1

Ingredients:

- 1/4cup onion

- 1 tomato

- 2 limes juice

- 1 avocado

- 1/4 teaspoon salt

- black pepper

- 1 jalapeno

- 1lb shrimp

- 1tablespoon cilantro

Directions:

1. Mix onion, lime juice, salt and pepper leave within 5 minutes. In another bowl, add chopped shrimp, avocado, tomato, jalapeno and onion mixture. Put salt and pepper, toss and serve.

Nutrition:

Calories: 365

Carbs: 15g

Fat: 17g

Protein: 25g

30.   Smoky Cauliflower Bites

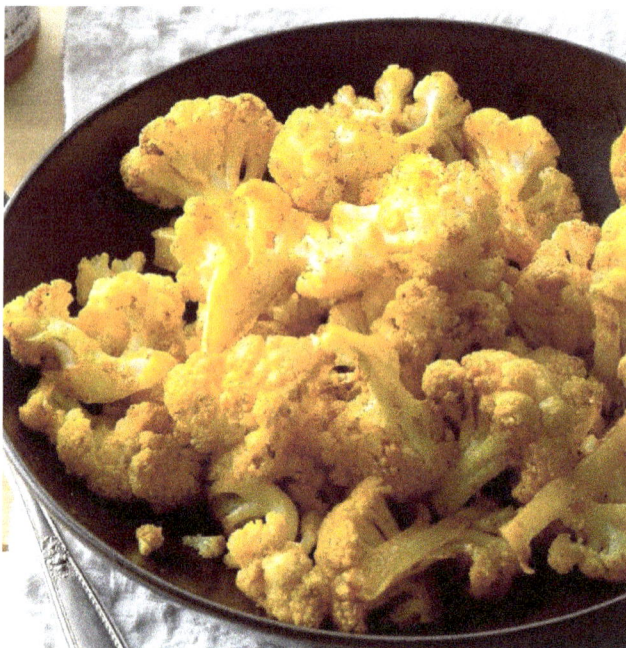

Preparation Time: 15 minutes

Cooking Time: 25 minutes

Servings: 2

Ingredients:

- 1 cauliflower

- 2 garlic cloves

- 2tablespoon olive oil

- 2tablespoon parsley

- 1teaspoon paprika

- 3/4teaspoon salt

Directions:

1. Mix cauliflower, olive oil, paprika and salt. Warm-up oven at 450. Bake within 10 minutes. Put garlic and bake within 10 to 15 minutes. Serve with parsley.

Nutrition:

Calories: 69

Carbs: 8g

Fat: 3g

Protein: 1g

DINNER

31.   Keto Lasagna

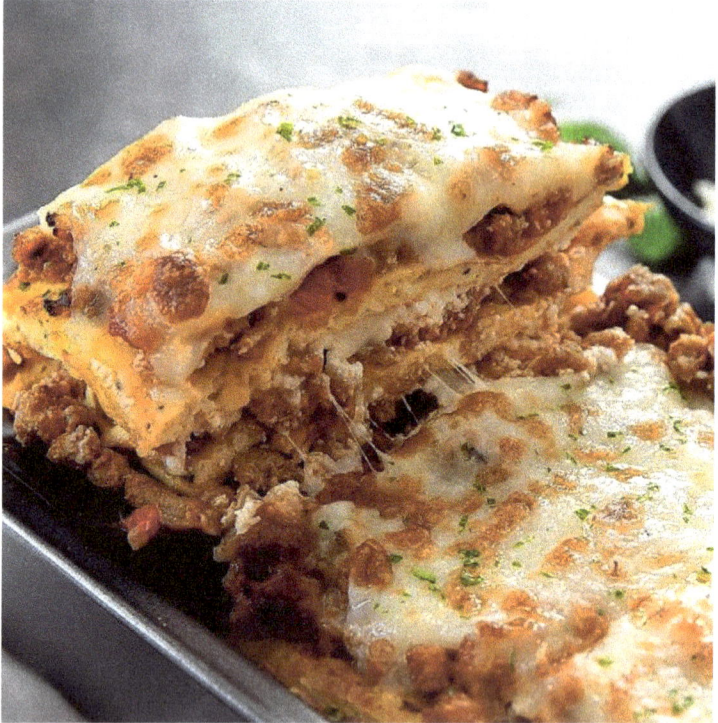

Preparation time: 15 minutes

Cooking time: 1 hour

Servings: 2

Ingredients:

- 8oz. block cream cheese

- 3 eggs

- Kosher salt

- Ground black pepper
- 2cups mozzarella
- ½cup parmesan
- Pinch red pepper flakes
- parsley
- Sauce:
- ¾cup marinara
- 1tablespoon. tomato paste
- 1lb. ground beef
- ½cup parmesan
- 1.5cup mozzarella
- 1tablespoon. extra virgin olive oil
- 1teaspoon. dried oregano
- 3 cloves garlic
- ½cup onion
- 16oz. ricotta

Directions:

1. Warm-up oven to 350 degrees.
2. Melt in the cream cheese, mozzarella, and parmesan. Put the eggs, salt and pepper.
3. Bake for 15 to 20 minutes.

4. Cook the onion within 5 minutes, then the garlic. Put the tomato paste. Add the ground beef, put salt and pepper. Cook then put aside.

5. Cook marinara sauce, put pepper, red pepper flakes, and ground pepper. Stir.

6. Take out the noodles and cut in half widthwise and then cut them again into 3 pieces.

7. Put 2 noodles at the bottom of the dish, then layer the parmesan and mozzarella shreds alternately.

8. Bake within 30 minutes. Garnish and serve.

Nutrition:

Calories: 508

Carbs: 8g

Fat: 39g

Protein: 33g

32. Creamy Tuscan Garlic Chicken

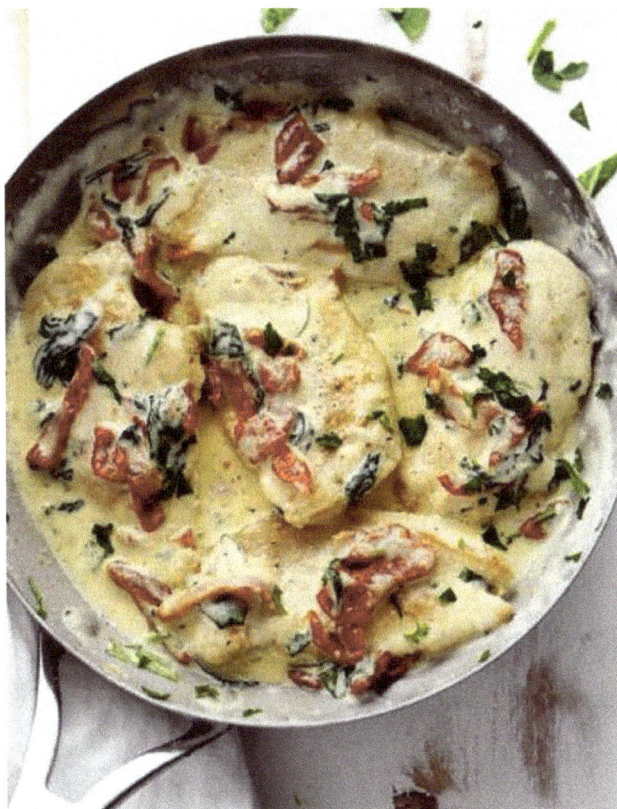

Preparation time: 15 minutes

Cooking time: 30 minutes

Servings: 4

Ingredients:

1.5 pounds chicken breast

½cup chicken broth

½cup parmesan cheese

½cup sun-dried tomatoes

1cup heavy cream

1cup spinach

2tablespoon. olive oil

1teaspoon. garlic powder

1teaspoon. Italian seasoning

Directions:

Cook the chicken using olive oil, medium heat within 5 minutes, put aside.

Combine the heavy cream, garlic powder, Italian seasoning, parmesan cheese, and chicken broth. Add the sundried tomatoes and spinach and simmer. Add the chicken back and serve.

Nutrition:

Calories: 368

Carbs: 7g

Fat: 0g

Protein: 30g

33. Ancho Macho Chili

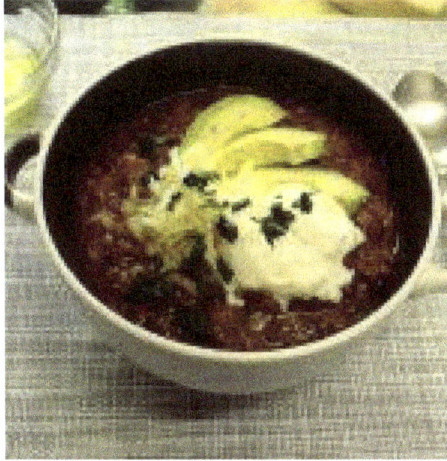

Preparation Time: 20 minutes

Cooking Time: 1 hour and 30 minutes

Servings: 4

Ingredients:

- 2lbs. lean sirloin

- Salt 1teaspoon

- Pepper 0.25teaspoon

- Olive Oil 1.5tablespoons

- Onion

- Chili Powder

- 7oz can tomato with green chilis

- ½cup chicken broth

- 2cloves garlic

Directions:

1. Warm-up oven to a temperature of 350F. Coat beef with pepper and salt.

2. Cook a third of the beef. Cook the onion for a few minutes. Put in the last four ingredients and simmer. Add in the beef with all its juices and cook within two hours. Stir and serve.

Nutrition:

Net carbs: 6g

Fat: 40g

Protein: 58g

Calories: 644kcal

34. Chicken Supreme Pizza

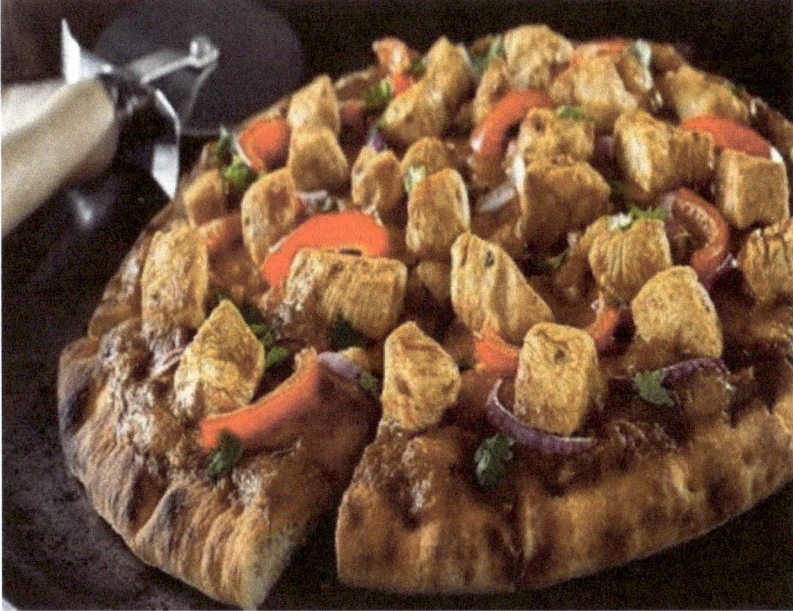

Preparation Time: 25 minutes

Cooking Time: 30 minutes

Servings: 4-8

Ingredients:

- 5oz cooked chicken breast
- Almond Flour 1.5cups
- Baking Powder 1teaspoon
- Salt half-teaspoon
- Water 0.25 cup
- Red Onion 1
- Red Pepper 1

- Green Pepper

- Mozzarella Cheese 1cup

- Olive Oil 3tablespoons

Directions:

1. Warm-up oven to a temperature of 400F.

2. Blend the flour both the salt and baking powder. Put the water and the oil added to the flour mixture to make the dough. Flattened dough.

3. Dump out the dough. Press it out, and coat the pan with oil.

4. Bake within 12 minutes. Remove then sprinkle with cheese and then add chicken, pepper, and onion. Bake again within 15 minutes, slice and serve.

Nutrition:

Net carbs: 4g

Fiber: 10g

Fat: 12g

Protein: 16g

Calories: 310kcal

35. Baked Jerked Chicken

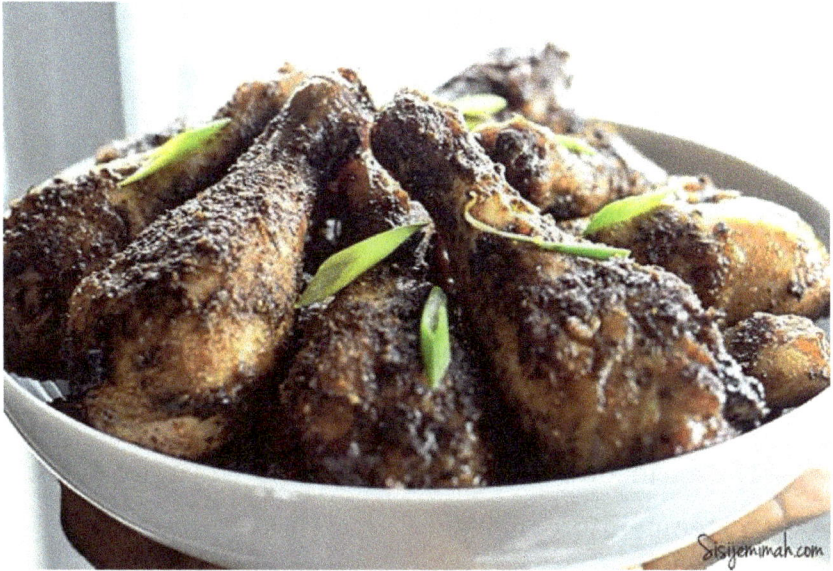

Preparation Time: 20 minutes

Cooking Time: 1 hour and 30 minutes

Servings: 4

Ingredients:

- 2pounds chicken thighs
- Olive Oil 0.33 cup
- Apple Cider Vinegar
- Salt 1teaspoon
- Powdered Onion 1teaspoon
- garlic half-teaspoon
- Nutmeg half-teaspoon

- Pepper half-teaspoon

- Powdered Ginger half-teaspoon

- Powdered Cayenne half-teaspoon

- Cinnamon 0.25 teaspoon

- Dried Thyme 0.25 teaspoon

Directions:

1. Mix all fixing, excluding the chicken. Stir in the prepared chicken pieces. Stir well.

2. Marinade within 4 hours. Warm-up oven to a temperature of 375F.

3. Cook within 1.25 hours. Adjust to broil chicken within 4 minutes. Serve.

Nutrition:

Net carbs: 4g

Fiber: 0g

Fat: 12g

Protein: 16g

Calories: 185kcal

36. Chicken Schnitzel

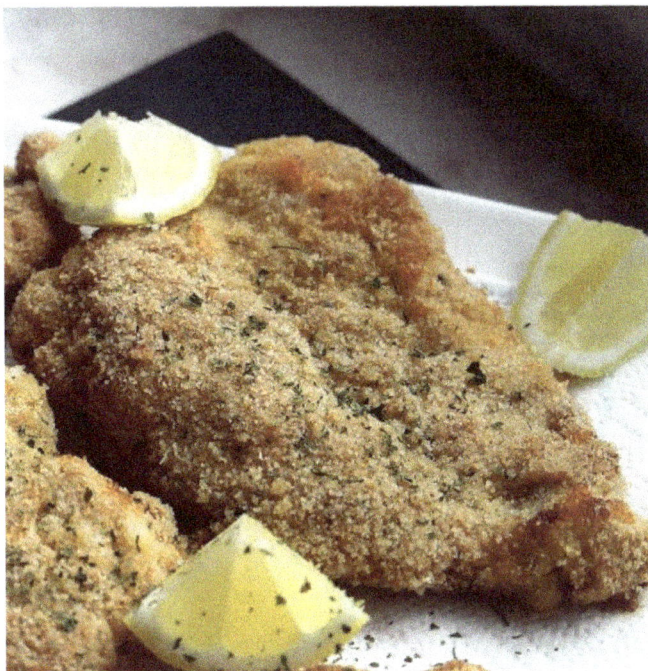

Preparation Time: 15 minutes

Cooking Time: 15 minutes

Servings: 3

Ingredients:

1. 1-pound chicken breast

2. Almond Flour 0.5 cups

3. Egg 1

4. Powdered Garlic half-tablespoon

5. A powdered onion a half-tablespoon

6. Keto-Safe Oil

7. **Directions:**

8. Combine the garlic power flour and onion in a bowl. Separately, beat the egg.

9. With a mallet, pound out the chicken. Put the chicken in the egg mixture. Then roll well through the flour.

10. Take a deep-frying pan and warm-up the oil to medium-high temperature.

11. Add chicken in batches. Fry. Pat dry and serve.

Nutrition:

Net carbs: 32g

Fiber: 0g

Fat: 17g

Protein: 61g

Calories: 541kcl

37. Broccoli and Chicken Casserole

Preparation Time: 15 minutes

Cooking Time: 10 minutes

Servings: 4

Ingredients:

1 ½ lb. chicken breast

8 oz softened cream cheese

Heavy Cream 0.5 cups

Powdered Garlic 1 teaspoon

Powdered Onion 1 teaspoon

Salt half-teaspoon

Pepper half-teaspoon

Broccoli 2 cups, florets

Mozzarella 1 cup

Parmesan 1 cup

Directions:

Warm-up oven to a temperature of 400F.

Combine the cream cheese to pepper and salt. Stir in the cubed chicken.

Put in the baking dish. Put the broccoli into the chicken-cheese mixture.

Top the dish with cheese, bake about 26 minutes and remove. Take off the foil and bake again for 10 minutes. Serve.

Nutrition:

Net carbs: 20g

Fiber: 0g

Fat: 25g

Protein: 21g

Calories: 391kcal

38. Baked Fish with Lemon Butter

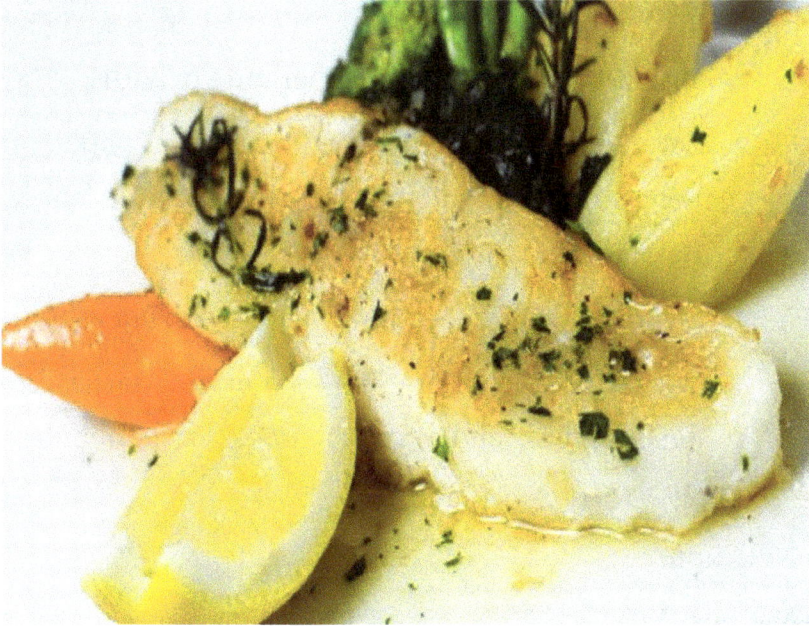

Preparation Time: 15 minutes

Cooking Time: 15 minutes

Servings: 2

Ingredients:

- 12 oz white fish fillets

- Olive Oil 1 tablespoon

- Pepper

- Salt

- Broccoli 1 medium-sized

- Butter 2 tablespoons

- Garlic Paste 1 teaspoon

- Lemon 1 medium-sized

Directions:

1. Warm-up the oven to a temperature of 430F.

2. Set the fish out onto the parchment paper, and put pepper and salt. Pour over olive oil and lemon slices. Bake within 15 minutes.

3. Steam the broccoli within five minutes. Put aside.

4. Warm-up, the butter, then stirs in zest, garlic, remaining lemon slices, and broccoli. Cook for 2 minutes before serving.

Nutrition:

Net carbs: 1g

Fiber: 0g

Fat: 15g

Protein: 34g

Calories: 276kcal

39. Chicken Broccoli Alfredo

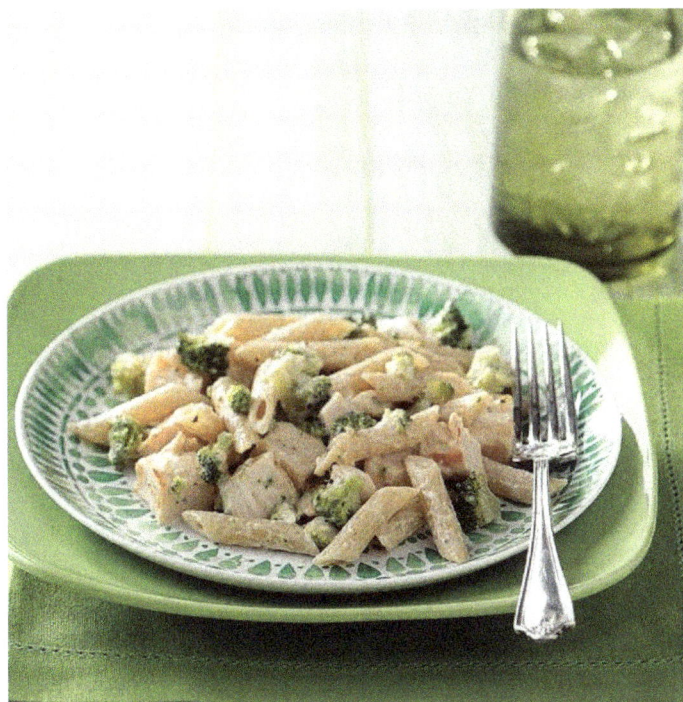

Preparation Time: 15 minutes

Cooking Time: 10 minutes

Servings: 4

Ingredients:

- Chicken Breast 1 pound

- Spinach 0.5 cups

- Broccoli 1 cup

- Butter 1 tablespoon

- Heavy Cream 0.5 cups

- Garlic 1 clove

- Chopped Onion 2 tablespoons

- ½ teaspoon of salt

- ½ teaspoon of pepper

Directions:

1. Boil broccoli within 10 minutes.

2. Melt the butter with onion and garlic, put the chicken. Sauté within 5 minutes.

3. Put the spinach and broccoli then stir in the cream with seasonings. Cook within 5 minutes and serve.

Nutrition:

Net carbs: 34g

Fiber: 0g

Fat: 19g

Protein: 34g

Calories: 523kcal

40. Grilled Cheesy Buffalo Chicken

Preparation Time: 15 minutes

Cooking Time: 10 minutes

Servings: 2

Ingredients:

- 10 oz chicken breast
- Garlic 2 cloves
- Mozzarella Cheese 0.25 cup
- Butter 1 tablespoon
- Hot Sauce 0.25 cup
- Lemon Juice 1 tablespoon
- Celery Salt 0.25 teaspoon
- Pepper
- salt

Directions:

1. Mix the minced garlic, hot sauce, celery salt, melted butter, lemon juice, pepper, and salt then put the chicken into the mixture.

2. Fill each chicken breast with cheese. Roll up, then secure with a toothpick to close the pocket.

3. Grease the grill. Cook within 5 minutes, flipping and do another 5 minutes. Nutrition:

Net carbs: 2g

Fiber: 1g

Fat: 5g

Protein: 24g

Calories: 150kcal

VEGETARIANS

41. Portobello Mushroom Pizza

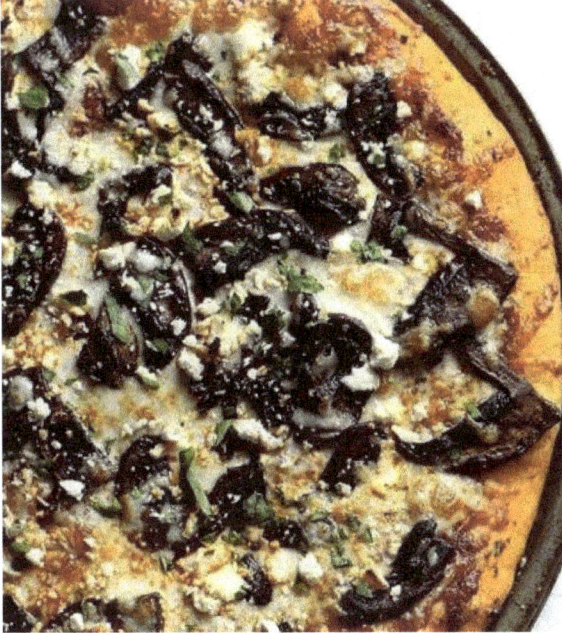

Preparation Time: 15 minutes

Cooking Time: 5 minutes

Servings: 4

Ingredients:

- 4 large portobello mushrooms, stems removed
- ¼ cup olive oil
- 1 teaspoon minced garlic
- 1 medium tomato, cut into 4 slices

- 2 teaspoons chopped fresh basil

- 1 cup shredded mozzarella cheese

Directions:

1. Preheat the oven to broil. Line a baking sheet with aluminum foil and set aside.

2. In a small bowl, toss the mushroom caps with the olive oil until well coated. Use your fingertips to rub the oil in without breaking the mushrooms.

3. Place the mushrooms on the baking sheet gill-side down and broil the mushrooms until they are tender on the tops, about 2 minute

4. Flip the mushrooms over and broil 1 minute more

5. Take the baking sheet out and spread the garlic over each mushroom, top each with a tomato slice, sprinkle with the basil, and top with the cheese

6. Broil the mushrooms until the cheese is melted and bubbly, about 1 minute.

7. Serve.

Nutrition:

Calories: 251

Fat: 20g

Protein: 14g

Carbs: 7g

Fiber: 3g

Net Carbs: 4g

Fat 71

Protein 19

Carbs 10

42. Garlicky Green Beans

Preparation Time: 10 minutes

Cooking Time: 10 minutes

Servings: 4

Ingredients:

- 1 pound green beans, stemmed
- 2 tablespoons olive oil
- 1 teaspoon minced garlic
- Sea salt
- Freshly ground black pepper
- ¼ cup freshly grated Parmesan cheese

Directions:

1. Preheat the oven to 425°F. Line a baking sheet with aluminum foil and set aside.

2. In a large bowl, toss together the green beans, olive oil, and garlic until well mixed.

3. Season the beans lightly with salt and pepper

4. Spread the beans on the baking sheet and roast them until they are tender and lightly browned, stirring them once, about 10 minutes.

5. Serve topped with the Parmesan cheese.

Nutrition:

Calories: 104

Fat: 9g

Protein: 4g

Carbs: 2g

Fiber: 1g

Net Carbs: 1g

Fat 77

Protein 15

Carbs 8

43. Sautéed Asparagus With Walnuts

Preparation Time: 10 minutes

Cooking Time: 5 minutes

Servings: 4

Ingredients:

- 1½ tablespoons olive oil

- ¾ pound asparagus, woody ends trimmed

- Sea salt

- Freshly ground pepper

- ¼ cup chopped walnuts

Directions:

1. Place a large skillet over medium-high heat and add the olive oil.

2. Sauté the asparagus until the spears are tender and lightly browned, about 5 minutes.

3. Season the asparagus with salt and pepper.

4. Remove the skillet from the heat and toss the asparagus with the walnuts.

5. Serve.

Nutrition:

Calories: 124

Fat: 12g

Protein: 3g

Carbs: 4g

Fiber: 2g

Net Carbs: 2g

Fat 81

Protein

Carbs 10

44. Brussels Sprouts Casserole

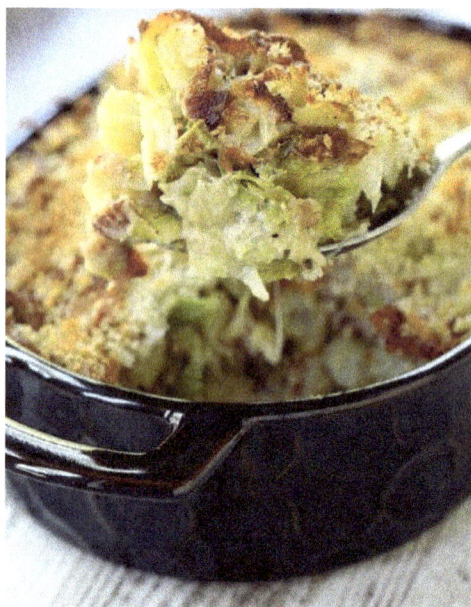

Preparation Time: 15 minutes

Cooking Time: 30 minutes

Servings: 8

Ingredients:

- 8 bacon slices

- 1 pound Brussels sprouts, blanched for 10 minutes and cut into quarters

- 1 cup shredded Swiss cheese, divided

- ¾ cup heavy (whipping) cream

Directions:

1. Preheat the oven to 400°F.

2. Place a skillet over medium-high heat and cook the bacon until it is crispy, about 6 minutes.

3. Reserve 1 tablespoon of bacon fat to grease the casserole dish and roughly chop the cooked bacon.

4. Lightly oil a casserole dish with the reserved bacon fat and set aside.

5. In a medium bowl, toss the Brussels sprouts with the chopped bacon and ½ cup of cheese and transfer the mixture to the casserole dish.

6. Pour the heavy cream over the Brussels sprouts and top the casserole with the remaining ½ cup of cheese.

7. Bake until the cheese is melted and lightly browned and the vegetables are heated through, about 20 minutes.

8. Serve.

Nutrition:

Calories: 299

Fat: 11g

Protein: 12g

Carbs: 7g

Fiber: 3g

Net Carbs: 4g

Fat 77

Protein 15 - Carbs 8

45. Creamed Spinach

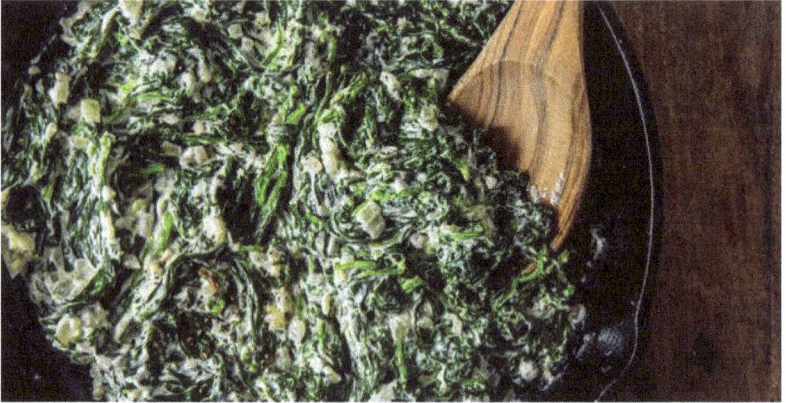

Preparation Time: 10 minutes

Cooking Time: 30 minutes

Servings: 4

Ingredients:

- 1 tablespoon butter

- ½ sweet onion, very thinly sliced

- 4 cups spinach, stemmed and thoroughly washed

- ¾ cup heavy (whipping) cream

- ¼ cup Herbed Chicken Stock (here)

- Pinch sea salt

- Pinch freshly ground black pepper

- Pinch ground nutmeg

Directions:

1. In a large skillet over medium heat, add the butter.

2. Sauté the onion until it is lightly caramelized, about 5 minutes.

3. Stir in the spinach, heavy cream, chicken stock, salt, pepper, and nutmeg.

4. Sauté until the spinach is wilted, about 5 minutes.

5. Continue cooking the spinach until it is tender and the sauce is thickened, about 15 minutes.

6. Serve immediately.

Nutrition:

Calories: 195

Fat: 20g

Protein: 3g

Carbs: 3g

Fiber: 2g

Net Carbs: 1g

Fat 88

Protein 6

Carbs 6

46. Cheesy Mashed Cauliflower

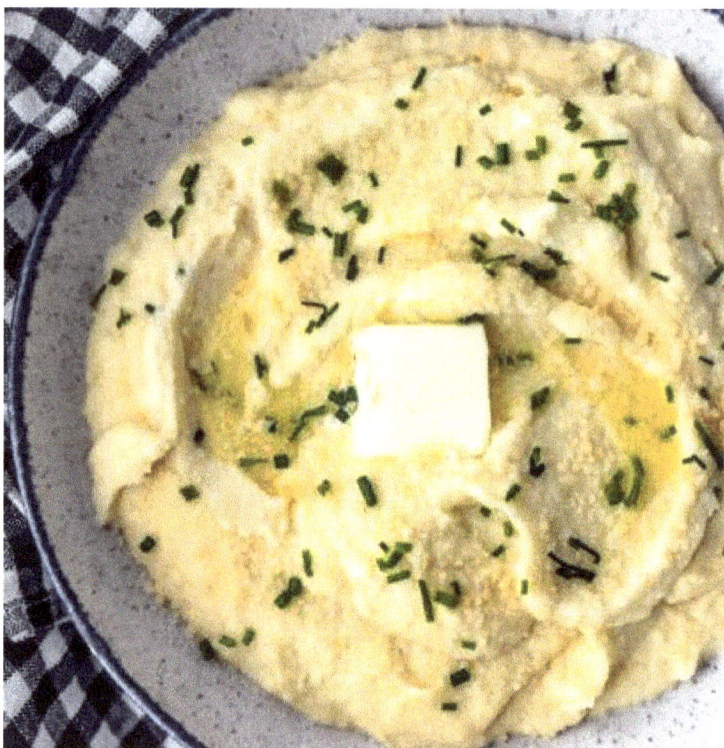

Preparation Time: 15 minutes

Cooking Time: 5 minutes

Servings: 4

Ingredients:

- 1 head cauliflower, chopped roughly

- ½ cup shredded Cheddar cheese

- ¼ cup heavy (whipping) cream

- 2 tablespoons butter, at room temperature

- Sea salt

- Freshly ground black pepper

Directions:

1. Place a large saucepan filled three-quarters full with water over high heat and bring to a boil.

2. Blanch the cauliflower until tender, about 5 minutes, and drain.

3. Transfer the cauliflower to a food processor and add the cheese, heavy cream, and butter. Purée until very creamy and whipped.

4. Season with salt and pepper.

5. Serve.

Nutrition:

Calories: 183

Fat: 15g

Protein: 8g

Carbs: 6g

Fiber: 2g

Net Carbs: 4g

Fat 75

Protein 14

Carbs 11

47. Sautéed Crispy Zucchini

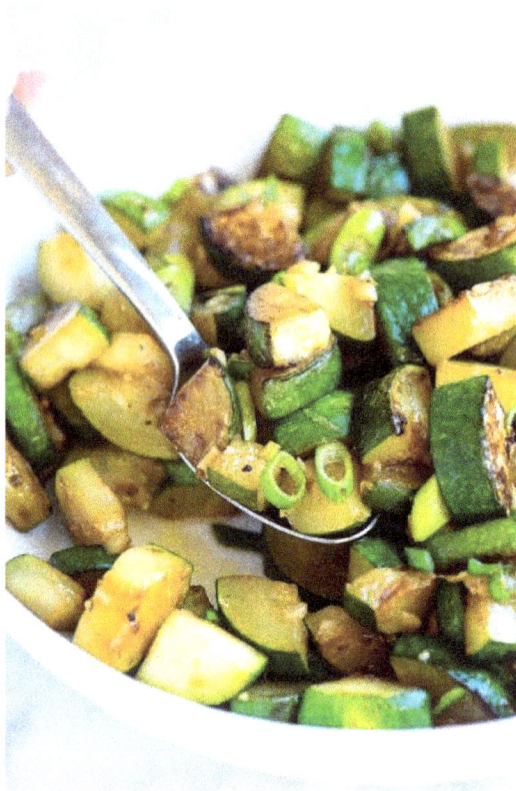

Preparation Time: 15 minutes

Cooking Time: 10 minutes

Servings: 4

Ingredients:

- 2 tablespoons butter

- 4 zucchini, cut into ¼-inch-thick rounds

- ½ cup freshly grated Parmesan cheese

- Freshly ground black pepper

Directions:

1. Place a large skillet over medium-high heat and melt the butter.

2. Add the zucchini and sauté until tender and lightly browned, about 5 minutes.

3. Spread the zucchini evenly in the skillet and sprinkle the Parmesan cheese over the vegetables.

4. Cook without stirring until the Parmesan cheese is melted and crispy where it touches the skillet, about 5 minutes.

5. Serve.

Nutrition:

Calories: 94

Fat: 8g

Protein: 4g

Carbs: 1g

Fiber: 0g

Net Carbs: 1g

Fat 76

Protein 20

Carbs 4

48.   Mushrooms With Camembert

Preparation Time: 5 minutes

Cooking Time: 15 minutes

Servings: 4

Ingredients:

- 2 tablespoons butter

- 2 teaspoons minced garlic

- 1 pound button mushrooms, halved

- 4 ounces Camembert cheese, diced

- Freshly ground black pepper

Directions:

1. Place a large skillet over medium-high heat and melt the butter.

2. Sauté the garlic until translucent, about 3 minutes.

3. Sauté the mushrooms until tender, about 10 minutes.

4. Stir in the cheese and sauté until melted, about 2 minutes.

5. Season with pepper and serve.

Nutrition:

Calories: 161

Fat: 13g

Protein: 9g

Carbs: 4g

Fiber: 1g

Net Carbs: 3g

Fat 70

Protein 21

Carbs 9

49. Pesto Zucchini Noodles

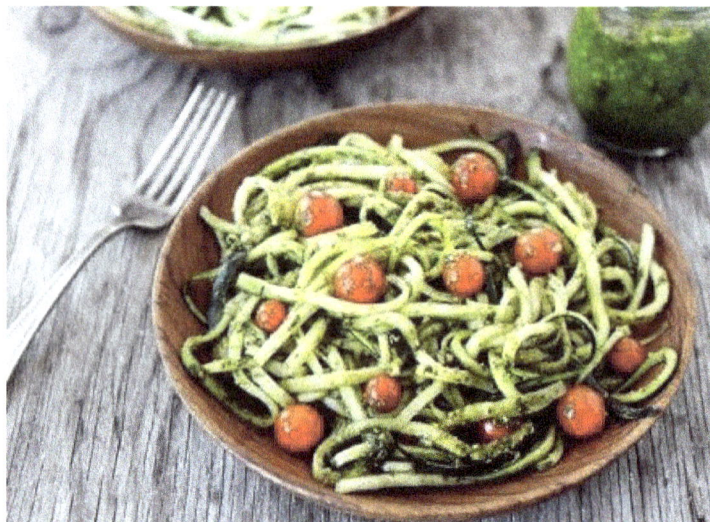

Preparation Time: 15 minutes

Cooking Time: 10 minutes

Servings: 4

Ingredients:

- 4 small zucchini, ends trimmed
- ¾ cup Herb Kale Pesto (here)¼ cup grated or shredded
- Parmesan chees

Directions:

1. Use a spiralizer or peeler to cut the zucchini into "noodles" and place them in a medium bowl.

2. Add the pesto and the Parmesan cheese and toss to coat.

3. Serve.

Nutrition:

Calories: 93

Fat: 8g

Protein: 4g

Carbs: 2g

Fiber: 0g

Net Carbs: 2g

Fat 70

Protein 15

Carbs 8

50. Golden Rosti

Preparation Time: 15 minutes

Cooking Time: 15 minutes

Servings: 8

Ingredients:

- 8 bacon slices, chopped
- 1 cup shredded acorn squash
- 1 cup shredded raw celeriac
- 2 tablespoons grated or shredded Parmesan cheese
- 2 teaspoons minced garlic
- 1 teaspoon chopped fresh thyme
- Sea salt
- Freshly ground black pepper
- 2 tablespoons butter

Directions:

1. In a large skillet over medium-high heat, cook the bacon until crispy, about 5 minutes.

2. While the bacon is cooking, mix together the squash, celeriac, Parmesan cheese, garlic, and thyme in a large bowl. Season the mixture generously with salt and pepper, and set aside.

3. Remove the cooked bacon with a slotted spoon to the rosti mixture and stir to incorporate.

4. Remove all but 2 tablespoons of bacon fat from the skillet and add the butter

5. Reduce the heat to medium-low and transfer the rosti mixture to the skillet and spread it out evenly to form a large round patty about 1 inch thick.

6. Cook until the bottom of the rosti is golden brown and crisp, about 5 minutes.

7. Flip the rosti over and cook until the other side is crispy and the middle is cooked through, about 5 minutes more.

8. Remove the skillet from the heat and cut the rosti into 8 pieces

9. Serve.

Nutrition:

Calories: 171

Fat: 15g

Protein: 5g

Carbs: 3g

Fiber: 0g

Net Carbs: 3g

Fat 81

Protein 12 - Carbs 7

CPSIA information can be obtained
at www.ICGtesting.com
Printed in the USA
LVHW080810220221
679596LV00025B/1270

9 781801 767682